Three Steps: Track, Manage Type 2 Diabetes & Prevent Complications!

Samya Boxberger-Oberoi,
Holistic Practitioner
&
Sandra Rajoo Gavney,
Registered Nurse

Three Steps: Track, Manage Type 2 Diabetes & Prevent Complications!

Foreword

I am glad Mrs. Samya Boxberger-Oberoi, a holistic practitioner in the US, and Mrs. Sandra Rajoo Gavney, a registered nurse, have written this book, *Three Steps: Track, Manage Type 2 Diabetes & Prevent Complications!,* which is the need of the hour. It is estimated that this disease worldwide afflicts 422 million people with Type 2 Diabetes being the most prevalent form.

The incidence of this disease has reached alarming numbers. With the deficiency of endocrinologists and general physicians, it has become necessary to complement the treating doctors with holistic practitioners and nursing care, especially for those suffering from Type 2 diabetes complications.

This book will immensely help medical practitioners to address this disease holistically and systematically. It will also provide patients with the necessary education about their condition and awareness to put in the much-needed effort to treat their condition. Most importantly, this work has been carefully done to achieve a sense of physical, mental, and social well-being as defined by the World Health Organization (WHO)'s mission statement.

The companion diary, which can be acquired separately, is a tool to record all activities and investigations required to monitor and continuously review the treatment towards managing the essential parameters of blood pressure, blood sugar, and cholesterol thereby restoring the most important factors affecting health and a feeling of wellness amongst patients with Type 2 diabetes.

The suggested holistic approach towards the treatment of this condition by treating doctors and a support team will bring comfort to the afflicted world population and enable them to live a happy and healthy life by mitigating complications associated with the disease, which include *diapression*, diabetes-related depression, nerve and blood vessel damage, blindness, kidney damage, coronary artery disease, foot damage, hearing impairment, Alzheimer's disease, gum and skin diseases.

Managed holistically and systematically as outlined in the book, we hope to manage the disease, which at present is a lifetime condition. I commend the authors for their effort and work. I am hopeful the book, and its companion will find use with every patient and the medical fraternity engaged in treating patients with Type 2 diabetes.

Dr. N. Bhardwaj, M.D

Acknowledgments

We are grateful to Dr. Narottam Bhardwaj for sharing his medical expertise with us, which spans more than forty years, and the validation of our work. A 1973 graduate of Maulana Azad Medical College New Delhi and a 1978 post-graduate in medicine from the same institution, Dr. Bhardwaj practices internal medicine. He is an expert on diabetes, a member of the Delhi Medical Association and the American Diabetic Association.

We are thankful and appreciative of the support we have received from our spouses, family members, friends, and those who routinely place their care and trust in us. Type 2 Diabetes, the most prevalent form of the disease and the primary topic of this book, has truly become a global pandemic. With their support and continuous encouragement, we are hopeful that we have done our part to provide our readers with the education and tools needed to manage their condition.

Table of Contents

Introduction

This book aims to promote health and wellbeing, as per the World Health Organization (WHO) guiding principles, which defines health as "a state of complete physical, mental, social well-being and not merely the absence of disease or infirmity."[1]

To that effect, the book offers a holistic framework for tracking, managing Type 2 diabetes, and preventing complications. This approach has become necessary to deliver the best results. It involves actively keeping track of all your daily activities and investigations for referencing by your doctors from time-to-time. It also requires a support system as given in this book, which includes trusted friend(s), family member(s), doctor(s), and other health professionals.

A holistic approach takes into consideration your physical, mental and emotional health, and social factors that may affect those. Teaming up with a holistic practitioner, who will coordinate the management of your condition with members of your support system, is vital to delivering the requisite care. It is to be understood from this point forward that managing the essentials parameters (blood sugar, blood pressure, and cholesterol) requires also proper management of stress and lifestyle factors apart from medications.

---

[1] The Constitution was adopted by the International Health Conference held in New York from 19 June to 22 July 1946, signed on 22 July 1946 by the representatives of 61 States (Off. Rec. Wld Hlth Org., 2, 100), and entered into force on 7 April 1948. Amendments adopted by the Twenty-sixth, Twenty-ninth, Thirty-ninth and Fifty-first World Health Assemblies (resolutions WHA26.37, WHA29.38, WHA39.6 and WHA51.23) came into force on 3 February 1977, 20 January 1984, 11 July 1994 and 15 September 2005 respectively and are incorporated in the present text. ("Constitution." World Health Organization, World Health Organization, www.who.int/about/who-we-are/constitution).

The management of your care will otherwise fall on you, a family member and/or a caregiver, who may not have the time, knowledge or understanding of the big picture to ensure optimal care. Similarly, without a support system in place, tackling your condition on your own may become overwhelming. Understandably, managing this condition requires daily monitoring, frequent communication with health professionals, scheduling of recurring medical examination, diagnostic tests, follow-up visits, and a protocol of healthy habits.

A diary to log all your activities, including all you eat, the medications and time when administered, and any form of physical activity performed daily is an ideal tool for subsequent referencing. It will enable you to make the needed lifestyle changes, to manage your sugar levels, and with the help of your team, to delay, mitigate and/or prevent the onset of complications. The same diary, which makes it possible for you to record this information, is of utmost importance for accurate and meaningful conversations with your doctor(s).

Your doctor(s) can work with you to bring your Type 2 diabetes under control if you follow the guidelines as outlined in this book. Your condition cannot be solely managed by medications; external factors, such as obesity and emotional stress, are linked to pre-diabetes and remain prevalent amongst Type 2 diabetics. Your doctor(s) can help identify the external factors and triggers that affect your condition. Do not forget to you do your part to acknowledge and face those as well. Other professionals can assist.

Almost one-fourth of the world population is afflicted by this condition, with an equal number of pre-diabetics (potential diabetics). In recent decades, obesity has struck humanity like a Tsunami. It is a major risk factor for pre-diabetes, a condition preventable through lifestyle changes, and a protocol of healthy eating, physical activity, and stress management. Left unchecked, this same condition most probably will lead to Type 2 diabetes, a lifetime condition. In 2015, the number of pre-diabetics in the U.S. population exceeded that of diabetics:

- An estimated 84.1 million aged 18 or older, or 33.9 % of U.S. population, were pre-diabetics;
- An estimated 30.3 million people of all ages, or 9.4% of the US population, were diabetics;
- 90% to 95% of all diabetes cases were Type 2 diabetes.[2]

With such alarming numbers, it has become essential to apply a holistic approach to deal with the menace. Aside from obesity, emotional stress is another major risk factor. Emotional stress results in hormonal imbalance, increased blood sugar levels, fatigue, and beta-cell dysfunction and insulin resistance. Stress, present in daily lifestyle, feeling overwhelmed and alone, all contribute to increasing your risk of suffering from depression, which can aggravate your condition. Because "diabetes can put a person at a greater risk of depression," it is important to discuss signs of distress such as loss of interest, feeling depressed, and irritability amongst other things with your doctor(s).[3]

Managing emotional stress, which causes glucose to pile up in your blood, is as important as keeping track of your daily eating habits and medication. Stress causes the body to react in fight-or-flight response mode that triggers the release of several hormones, which have the net effect of making stored energy – glucose and fat – available to cells raise blood sugar levels.[4]

---

[2] "National Diabetes Statistics Report | Data & Statistics | Diabetes | CDC." *Centers for Disease Control and Prevention*, Centers for Disease Control and Prevention, www.cdc.gov/diabetes/data/statistics-report/index.html.
[3] "Depression." *American Diabetes Association*, www.diabetes.org/living-with-diabetes/complications/mental-health/depression.html.
[4] "Stress." *American Diabetes Association*, www.diabetes.org/living-with-diabetes/complications/mental-health/stress.html.

Behavioral changes such as increased physical activity, mindful eating habits to lose weight if overweight or obese, breathing techniques and meditation, and partaking in your favorite hobbies such as music, and family activities will help you live life happily and joyously. This will contribute to reducing your emotional and physical stress.

Before you start your journey, it is important to work out a support system. This will ensure that you can monitor your progress scientifically. Your support system should include depending on your condition:

Trusted friend (s) & Family_____,
for moral and emotional support
Dr. _____, Endocrinologist (diabetes specialist)
Dr._____, Primary care physician
Dr. _____, Cardiologist
Dr._____, Neurologist
Dr_____, Nephrologist
Dr._____, Optometrist and/or ophthalmologist
Dr. _____, Psychiatrist
Dr. _____, Psychologist
Dr. _____, Podiatrist
Dr. _____, Dentist

A holistic approach may require the help of additional professionals, who can help you to follow through with your goals and offer other services that complement the care you are currently receiving. A dietician or nutritionist can be one of them to plan healthy meals, lose weight, while a holistic practitioner can coordinate your care and provide other services as well.

For best results, your condition should be managed holistically with a customized solution. Such an effort is provided by a holistic practitioner. Your role is to move forward to seek out the best possible care for yourself, to make use of all available resources to you, and to manage your condition to delay, mitigate and/or prevent complications. This is hard to achieve alone. You must enlist the help of others.

You can nonetheless keep track of all daily activities pertinent to your condition, monitoring of your blood sugar and blood pressure, taking medications if required, following up on all appointments, and implementing the recommended lifestyle changes and a protocol of healthy habits to name the essentials.

This book has a companion diary for recording the daily activities and investigations that affect individuals with your condition. The same diary is essentially to be employed by you and medical practitioners to carry out a systematic review of your condition as part of a holistic patient care management plan.

The Companion Diary to Three Steps: Track, Manage Type 2 Diabetes & Prevent Complications! is available for purchase from Amazon and other distribution channels.

Disclaimer: The content of this book and companion diary are not intended to be a substitute for professional medical advice, diagnosis, or treatment. Always seek the advice of your endocrinologist, physician or other qualified health provider with any questions you may have regarding your condition. Never disregard professional medical advice or delay in seeking it because of something you have read in these books. The authors are not responsible for any specific health needs and are not liable for any damages or negative consequences from any treatment, to any person reading or following the information in these books. Links to websites and reference to other publications are provided on an "as is" basis for informational and educational purposes. The authors have no control over the content published or claims made by these websites or publications. You are responsible for your own choices, actions, and results.

Your Support System

Your support system may be comprised of trusted friend(s), family member(s), medical practitioners and health professionals, and customized as per your condition. The table provides an overview of the roles and responsibilities of those who may be part of your team. This overview does not constitute a description of the scope of practice of each. This is for reference only.

Support Team	Role & Responsibilities
Trusted friend(s) and family	Provides moral and emotional support. May assist in other ways such as providing transportation, organizing outings, going for a walk, etc.
Caregiver, hired help or family member	Assists with the management of some, or all, aspects of care. May accompany to doctor visits, oversee the care of a loved one per care plan or provide care as instructed by the family and medical team.
Endocrinologist (i.e. a diabetes specialist)	Specializes in the glands of the endocrine system. The pancreas belongs to the endocrine and digestive systems. It produces hormones, notably insulin. Diabetics have a problem with making insulin or how their body uses insulin.
Primary care physician	Specializes in family medicine, internal medicine or pediatrics; provides initially care as the point of the first contact and takes responsibility for providing continuous care to the patient.
Cardiologist	Specializes in the study or treatment of heart diseases and heart abnormalities.

Neurologist	Specializes in treating diseases of the nervous system, which includes the brain and spinal cord.
Nephrologist	Specializes in kidney health and kidney disease.
Optometrist	Examines the eyes for visual defects and prescribes corrective lenses.
Ophthalmologist	Specializes in the study and treatment of disorders and diseases of the eye.
Psychiatrist	Specializes in the diagnosis and treatment of mental illness.
Psychologist	Provides counseling, help clients make behavioral changes, identify and diagnose mental, behavioral, or emotional disorders.
Podiatrist	Treats the feet and their ailments.
Dentist	Treats diseases and conditions that affect the teeth, gums and mouth; examines and performs routine cleaning, repairs teeth, extracts and inserts artificial ones.
Notes:	

A Holistic Practitioner

A holistic practitioner can work with you to create a customized solution and an individualized care plan. The purpose of the care plan is to manage your condition and organize aspects of your care requiring primarily your attention such as close monitoring of your daily activities, stress management, nutrition, and physical activities versus those requiring coordination with your care team to deliver the best possible results. The individualized care plan that your holistic practitioner will create with you, the lifestyle changes that you choose to work on and the medical care you received should all aim to keep your condition under control to manage your Type 2 diabetes, and delay, mitigate, and/or prevent complications.

Depending on your condition and needs, a holistic practitioner may provide:

- Education, support, and advocacy
- Deep dives into areas specific to your condition affecting your health and wellbeing
- Care management and client advocacy, i.e. a care plan, physician visit reports, etc.
- Coordination with your support team

The same practitioner may supplement the above with:

- Stress management, breathing, and relaxation techniques
- If appropriate, discuss the use of natural remedies (essential oils to support the above, e.g.)
- Discuss the benefits of physical activities and proper nutrition

Regardless of training, a holistic practitioner will focus on you as a whole person – body, mind, spirit, and emotions - with a quest for promoting wellbeing and health. A well-versed holistic practitioner has a good understanding of:

- Anatomy and physiology
- Nutrition and body chemistry
- Stress management, breathing, and relaxation techniques
- Allopathic (modern medicine) knowledge of your condition
- Well-researched complementary therapies such as therapeutic massages, yoga therapy, etc.
- Scholarly researched effects of traditional medicine, Chinese or Ayurveda
- Other complementary and alternative medicine (CAM)

A New Beginning!

The World Health Organization (WHO) currently estimates that 422 million people have diabetes worldwide.[5] Amongst them, 30.3 million Americans, or 9.4% of the US population.[6] These incidents are often the result of today's lifestyle and stress overload, whether it manifested physically, cognitively, emotionally, or behaviorally.

Diabetes, also known as diabetes mellitus, "is a chronic disease caused by inherited and/or acquired deficiency in production of insulin by the pancreas, or by the ineffectiveness of the insulin produced. Such a deficiency results in increased concentrations of glucose in the blood, which in turn damage many of the body's systems, in particular, blood vessels and nerves."[7]

The Mayo Clinic also describes this condition "as a group of diseases that affect how your body uses blood sugar (glucose). Glucose is vital to your health because it's an important source of energy for the cells that make up your muscles and tissues. It's also your brain's main source of fuel."[8]

Of all the forms of diabetes, Type 2 diabetes is the most prevalent form of the disease afflicting humanity. Many people are initially pre-diabetic and are not aware of it. Pre-diabetes is seen to be prevalent

---

[5] "Diabetes." *World Health Organization*, World Health Organization, www.who.int/news-room/fact-sheets/detail/diabetes.
[6] "New CDC Report: More than 100 Million Americans Have Diabetes or Prediabetes | CDC Online Newsroom | CDC." *Centers for Disease Control and Prevention*, Centers for Disease Control and Prevention, 18 July 2017, www.cdc.gov/media/releases/2017/p0718-diabetes-report.html.
[7] "Diabetes Mellitus." *World Health Organization*, World Health Organization, 22 Nov. 2010, www.who.int/mediacentre/factsheets/fs138/en/.
[8] "Diabetes." *Mayo Clinic*, Mayo Foundation for Medical Education and Research, 8 Aug. 2018, www.mayoclinic.org/diseases-conditions/diabetes/symptoms-causes/sys-20371444.

amongst younger people, especially amongst those who are obese. Pre-diabetes is a condition in a nascent stage that is potentially reversible with physical activity and diet control. It is estimated that at least 1 out of 3 Americans will develop diabetes in their lifetime, mostly Type 2 diabetes;[9] the net effect of pre-diabetes left unchecked.

The remainder of this book covers the most important facts about Type 2 diabetes, so that you can understand your condition and manage it adequately, including tracking and monitoring what is important, and how to best keep your condition under control. You will also find a table that contains a list of medical diagnostics and tests (Fact #13) related to your condition, a set of guidelines for diabetes (Fact #14), and a sample of a daily log at the end of this book.

The sample log is taken from The Companion Diary to *Three Steps: Track, Manage Type 2 Diabetes & Prevent Complications!* This companion diary allows you to record all daily activities and investigations for up to 12 weeks or 90 days. This practical and useful tool is not only handy for recording your daily vital signs, food and medication intake and activities but it is also helpful for monitoring and reviewing progress with your support system over 12 weeks. This period also coincides with the HbA1c quarterly monitoring of your blood sugar (glucose) average to see if those levels are stable and remain within range. The same HbA1c test is used to diagnose diabetes.[10]

---

[9] "National DPP Customer Service Center." *Centers for Disease Control and Prevention*, Centers for Disease Control and Prevention, www.nationaldppcsc.cdc.gov/s/article/CDC-2017-National-Diabetes-Statistics-Report-1525289365896.

[10] "Diagnosing Diabetes and Learning About Prediabetes." *American Diabetes Association*, www.diabetes.org/diabetes-basics/diagnosis/.

As you can see, we have done the work for you. The companion diary focuses merely on what is most relevant to you (after you are done with reading this book and consulting the additional resources therein), a short introduction and daily logs to record all activities and investigations necessary for you and your doctors to review your progress. The diary is available for purchase separately.

Fact #1 - You Are Not Alone!

The population afflicted by diabetes is on the rise worldwide. You are not alone. As previously stated, the World Health Organization estimates that 422 million suffer from diabetes in 2014, including 30.2 million Americans. Of all the types of diabetics, 90% of all diabetics in the US are suffering from Type 2 diabetes, which is often acquired in adulthood, [11] and can be well managed by following guidelines as outlined in this book.

All forms of diabetes can have an adverse effect on the body and organs. It is a chronic disease that gradually damages many of the body's systems, in particular, blood vessels and nerves,[12] and as such must be kept under control. In the form of Type 2, the condition can lead to a myriad of complications. Such complications not only include the nerve and vessel damage but may also lead to blindness, kidney failure, coronary artery disease (CAD), heart attacks, stroke, and/or lower limb amputation. If not kept under control, this condition can seriously impair the functioning of your kidneys and liver leading to life-threatening conditions.

A healthy diet, physical activity, maintaining a balanced bodyweight, managing stress, regular screening, and avoidance of junk food, consumption of alcohol and liquor, and most importantly, tobacco and sugar-based beverages are the essentials for delaying, mitigating and/or preventing complications associated with this condition.

Smoking and sugar-based beverages have the most deleterious effect of all on your condition. Smoking, specifically, is known to aggravate

---

[11] "Type 2 Diabetes | Basics | Diabetes | CDC." *Centers for Disease Control and Prevention*, Centers for Disease Control and Prevention, www.cdc.gov/diabetes/basics/type2.html.

[12] "Diabetes Mellitus." *World Health Organization,* World Health Organization, 22 Nor. 2010, www.who.int/mediacentre/factsheets/fs138/en/.

Type 2 diabetes and associated complications. If you smoke, make it a goal to quit. Apart from smoking, sugar-based beverages are already detrimental to the health of pre-diabetics and deadly for diabetes patients. Make it a goal to forgo both.

In this endeavor, the most important person is you. So, commit yourself without further procrastination to commence your journey today!

Fact #2 - Most Common Types of Diabetes

In the past, diabetes was classified into Type 1 and Type 2. There are at least five types of diabetes, with Type 2 being the most prevalent. A recent study published in *The Lancet Diabetes and Endocrinology Journal* in 2018 confirms these findings.

Today, it is well understood that Type 2 is lifestyle-related and develops progressively. As you age, it can significantly degrade your quality of life and prevent you from "aging gracefully." Continued high sugar levels manifest in coronary artery disease, high blood pressure, dementia, Alzheimer's, loss of eyesight, rheumatism, skin diseases, and a host of other complications.

Other types of diabetes such as Type 1, MODY, LADA as described in the article, *Types of Diabetes*, published by the Mayo clinic are generally not reversible and have to be managed through lifetime medications:

Type 1 is a rare autoimmune condition where the pancreas destroys cells responsible for producing insulin. Diabetics with Type 1 are dependent on insulin for life.

MODY, or maturity-onset diabetes of the young, is a hereditary and DNA related. It is caused by a gene mutation and often misdiagnosed as Type 1 or Type 2. The onset is before the age of 25. The pancreas does not produce enough insulin, which leads to a permanent diabetic condition.

LADA, or latent autoimmune diabetes in adults, is a slowly developing autoimmune Type 1 diabetes that occurs in adults. LADA eventually destroys the cells that produce insulin.

Gestational diabetes, in contrast, occurs during pregnancy. Generally, it resolves itself once the baby is born. It can increase the risk of developing Type 2 later on. [13]

So, what can you do?

As you are becoming more aware of your condition and its adverse effects on your body and organs, the time has come to work diligently with your support team as outlined in this book. This will allow you to enlist the help of your doctors and other professionals, who can provide the much-needed recommendations to manage your specific condition, bring your diabetes under control, and delay, mitigate and/or prevent complications.

Your holistic practitioner, if you have enlisted one, can work with you to coordinate with members of your team to deliver the best possible results. Your care plan will include your medical diagnoses, list of prescribed medication if applicable, and a protocol for a healthy diet, daily physical activity, weight balance; and, most importantly, strategies to manage stress and bring about emotional stability. So, take charge today!

While following the guidelines outlined in this book, remember that your commitment and efforts will go a long way to keep your condition under control, mitigate its adverse effects on your body and organs, or delay the onset of complications.

---

[13] "Types of Diabetes." *Services and Treatments - Mayo Clinic Health System*, 18 Oct. 2016, www.mayoclinichealthsystem.org/hometown-health/speaking-of-health/types-of-diabetes

Fact #3 - Benefits of Exercise and Diet

Medical science has proven that a lifestyle that includes diet and exercise plays a vital role in managing your Type 2 diabetes and other chronic health conditions.

Our goal here is to guide you in your journey to managing your condition, which is possible with lifestyle changes as simple as educating ourselves about your condition, its causes, complications, and manifestation in other serious conditions.

Let us start with the benefits of following a healthy diet. What are those?

Being overweight or obese is a condition that is prevalent amongst pre-diabetics and Type 2 diabetics. Maintenance of healthy and balanced weight can have a significant impact on your overall health. Reducing saturated fats found in meat proteins, reducing the consumption of dairy products and deep-fried foods can go a long way in reducing your body weight, belly fat, and attaining a normal Body Mass Index (BMI).

What about carbohydrates? How do they affect blood sugar levels?

There are two kinds of carbohydrates, simple and complex. Simple carbohydrates are digested quickly and are converted into sugar in our bloodstream. Complex carbohydrates are slowly digested, the better choice for optimal weight loss.

Simple carbohydrates are foods that contain sugars and starches that have been stripped of their natural fiber and nutrients. Complex carbohydrates are found in whole, unprocessed foods, including fruits, vegetables, legumes, and whole grains.

What about physical activity and an exercise protocol?

Being active physically is vital to your metabolism, immunity, and digesting what you eat. Initially, as little as 10 minutes of some form of daily workout can begin to have a positive impact on your health. An added benefit of exercising regularly is the ability of the body to release endorphins – a happy hormone that naturally brings about a feeling of wellness by reducing stress, pain, and preventing depression.

Regular exercise can ward off anxiety and depression, improves muscle tone, lowers blood pressure and blood sugar, helps reduce body fat, strengthens and builds bones, makes you look fit and healthy, and improves sleep to name a few.[14] In all, physical activity can enhance your quality of life and wellbeing. Talk to your endocrinologist, doctors, and support team. They can work with you towards achieving your goal.

---

[14] "Glossary." *Diabetes Education Online*, Diabetes Teaching Center at the University of California, San Francisco, www.dtc.ucsf.edu/types-of-diabetes/type2/.

Fact #4 – Testing and Monitoring

Consistency in daily testing and monitoring play an important part in achieving your goal to manage your condition and mitigate complications. This book describes what you should know and monitor daily overtime to share with your doctors, other health professionals, and your support team.

Any changes could indicate progress toward your goal, or a need for medication and diet review. Your endocrinologist can review these changes and help you reach the goals that you set for yourself. Some changes may initially be hard to detect and become more visible over time, which is why it is important to be consistent with testing, monitoring, and recording daily. Remember managing your condition requires patience; specifically, it involves:

- Testing three times daily if you are on insulin
- Daily, and as needed, if you are on an oral anti-diabetic medication

Make it a point to record these numbers and discuss those during medical appointments so that your doctors can provide the needed interventions to keep blood sugar, cholesterol, and blood pressure within the permissible limits.

It is a good idea to review your entries and to be reminded from time-to-time that uncontrolled diabetes is a serious health matter. Your condition can lead to a myriad of health complications, including nerve and blood vessel damage, high blood pressure, kidney disease or failure, loss of vision, coronary artery disease and diabetic ulcers to name a few. Keeping your blood sugar within a permissible range is an essential preventive measure against complications associated with diabetes.

When to test your blood sugar?

Test before having breakfast to know how much insulin to take, what you need to have for breakfast, and how much of your medication is needed. Follow your sliding scale for insulin intake as instructed by your doctor.

Do not run out of supplies such as insulin, strips, and lancets. Always have a one-week supply on hand, the same as for your oral medications. Watch out for symptoms of low blood sugar, known as hypoglycemia, and take steps to correct it immediately!

Monitor for symptoms of high blood sugar, known as hyperglycemia, as this may require hospitalization if not attended to.

You can find more information online about testing and monitoring. Remember education is key to the understanding of your condition and managing it adequately.

How to interpret your numbers?

The two tables below can help you to evaluate your numbers, discuss those with your support system, and your doctor(s). As outlined in this book, the Joslin Diabetes Center recommends that you use this information "as a guide to work with your doctor(s) and other health professionals to determine what your target goals should be and develop a program of regular blood glucose monitoring to manage your condition. "

The first table below shows the blood glucose ranges for diabetics and non-diabetics as published by Joslin Diabetes Center. Those ranges refer to your "plasma blood glucose range as opposed to the whole blood number," which is typically used by old glucometers. In general, "plasma number read about 10 - 12% higher than the older whole blood numbers. So, if your fasting and pre-meal blood glucose target is 90 - 130 mg/dl plasma glucose, it would be 80 - 120 mg/dl if your meter reads whole blood." [15]

When checking your numbers, keep the above in mind. If you have a new glucometer, your ranges will be aligned with those shown in this table. If you are using an older glucometer, consider the above variants.

Time of Check	Goal plasma blood glucose ranges for people without diabetes	Goal plasma blood glucose ranges for people with diabetes
Before breakfast (fasting)	< 100	70 – 130
Before lunch, dinner and snack	< 110	70 – 130
Two hours after meals	< 140	< 180
Bedtime	< 120	90- 150
A1c (also called glycosylated hemoglobin A1c, HbA1c, or glycohemoglobin A1c.)	< 6%	< 7%
Note: < = less than		

The second table shows the normal range for other values, vital signs. You should clarify these with your doctors and other health

[15] www.joslin.org, Joslin Diabetes Center. "Joslin Diabetes Center | Blood Glucose Chart." *Blood Glucose Chart | Joslin Diabetes Center*, www.joslin.org/info/Goals-for-Blood-Glucose-Control.html.

professionals as needed. The most important vital sign, in this case, for daily monitoring is your blood pressure.

120/80 mm Hg blood pressure is a normal average range. Blood pressure is typically higher for diabetics. Nonetheless, the American Diabetes Association "recommends a blood pressure target of less than 140/90 mm Hg for most people with diabetes and hypertension, a lower blood pressure goal might be beneficial for some patients who have a high risk of cardiovascular disease."[16]

Other Values / Vital Signs	
Blood Pressure	120/80 mm Hg
Body Temperature	98.2 to 98.7 Fahrenheit
Heart Rate	80 to 100 beats/min.
Oxygen Saturation	92+

---

[16] "American Diabetes Association Issues Updated Diabetes and Hypertension Position Statement." *American Diabetes Association*, www.diabetes.org/newsroom/press-releases/2017/american-diabetes-association-updated-diabetes-and-hypertension-position-statement-2017.html.

Fact #5 – Dietary Guidelines

A diabetic diet, along with physical activity and medications, is essential to help you manage your condition. Simply put, medical professionals and researchers have established guidelines to educate the community on evidence-based best practices and how to implement those for health benefits.

Following these dietary guidelines can not only improve your health, help mitigate complications, and assist in weight management but they can also help you develop a healthier relationship with food, which in turn will help you to make the best choice for yourself. A dietician or nutritionist can assist in designing healthy and enjoyable meal plans specific to your condition.

So, what are the guidelines a diabetic should follow?

- The best foods to eat
- The food and drinks to consume
- The portion sizes
- Carbohydrates tracking
- Reading labels

As a rule of thumb, the healthy fats to incorporate in your diet are fat from nuts, seeds, and avocados. These are the best choices. Avoid cooking with butter, margarine, vegetable oils, and other high saturated fats that have detrimental effects on your cholesterol, and health.

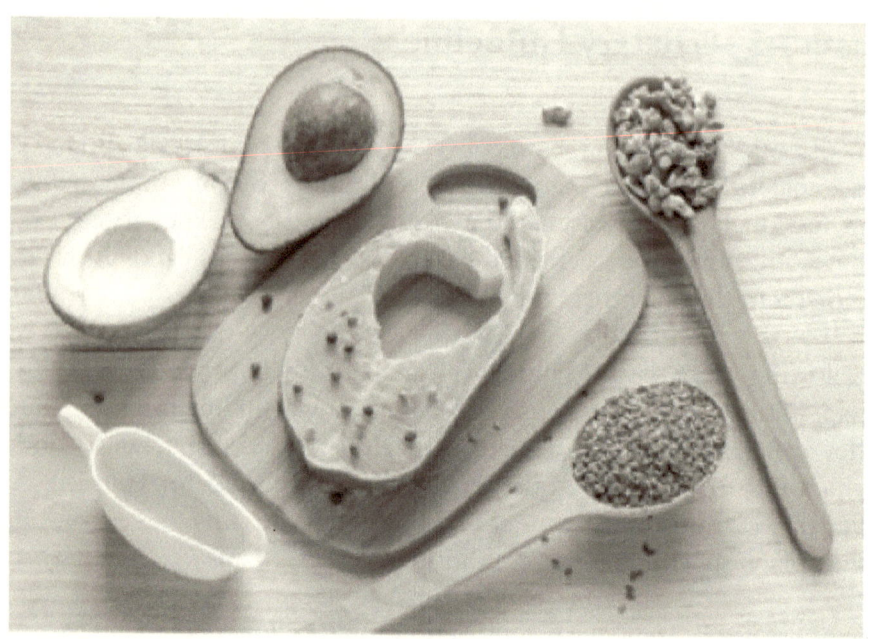

A balanced meal should include protein, grains, all color vegetables, fruits, and nuts. The right portions make up for a colorful and healthy dinner size plate with not too much or too little of the same types of foods. Have enough so you do not feel stuffed but satiated. A dietician or nutritionist can work with you to customize your diet to include all of the above and determine the correct portion sizes for your specific condition.

Many organizations published information relative to meal planning and interactive meal plans for diabetics on their website, including the American Diabetes Association, the Mayo Clinic, and the Joslin Diabetes Center. According to the Mayo Clinic, the American Diabetes Association has a set of simple, yet useful steps when preparing a plate:

- Fill half of your plate with non-starchy vegetables, such as spinach and tomatoes.

- Fill a quarter of your plate with a protein, such as tuna, lean pork or chicken.
- Fill the last quarter with a whole-grain item, such as brown rice, or a starchy vegetable, such as green peas.
- Include "good" fats such as nuts or avocados in small amounts.
- Add a serving of fruit or dairy and a drink of water or unsweetened tea or coffee.[17]

For a more interactive approach, try the Joslin's Healthy Plate. The interactive guide for healthy eating is a useful tool to customize your meals. As noted earlier and recommended by all, Joslin Diabetes Center also encourages diabetics to meet with a dietician to learn about meal planning and to develop an individualized eating plan.[18]

At the same time, make it a healthy habit to choose the right foods for you that are full of nutrients to keep you happy and healthy. Avoid eating processed foods and too many simple carbohydrates. Complex carbohydrates are a healthier choice!

---

[17] "Diabetes Diet: Create Your Healthy-Eating Plan." *Mayo Clinic*, Mayo Foundation for Medical Education and Research, 19 Feb. 2019, www.mayoclinic.org/diseases-conditions/diabetes/in-depth/diabetes-diet/art-20044295.
[18] www.joslin.org, Joslin Diabetes Center. "Diabetes & Nutrition." *Joslin Diabetes Center*, www.joslin.org/info/diabetes-and-nutrition.html.

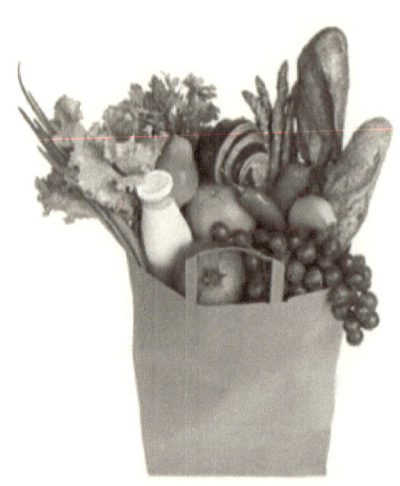

Your health is your wealth. Be rich with vitality and energy. Drink plenty of water and sugar-free drinks to keep your body fully hydrated. Apart from smoking, sugar-based beverages have a deleterious effect on pre-diabetics and are deadly to diabetics. Commit to forgo sugar-based drinks!

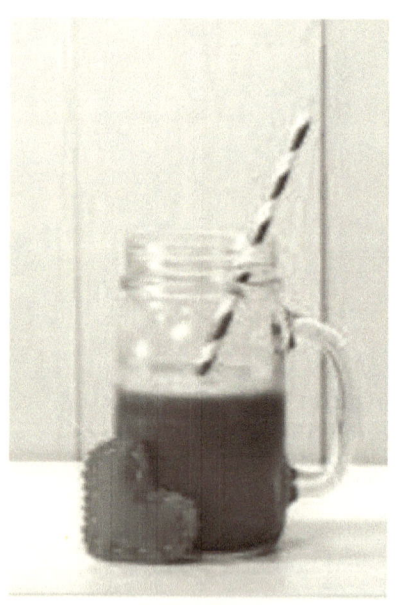

What about alcohol?

Fitting alcohol into your meal plan should be discussed with your doctors, other health professionals, and your support system.

Depending on your cultural background, "alcoholic beverages can be a common part of our social lives. Each adult must decide whether or not to use alcohol. When making this decision, you should understand what the potential effects of alcohol are on your health. Although alcohol has little effect on blood glucose control, it may worsen other medical problems. Make sure you discuss the use of alcohol with your doctor."[19]

Carefully reading all labels looking for hidden sugars such as high fructose corn syrup, cane sugar, agave, artificial and non-sweeteners is also extremely important, as these hidden sugars have a detrimental effect on your condition and associated complications.[20]

It is also a good idea to stay abreast of the latest food labeling requirements and regulations as those change from time-to-time. You can browse the internet to stay current and find out more information. As part of a healthier lifestyle, it is best to avoid certain condiments and/or eat other condiments in moderation. Some labels require extra scrutiny as some condiments contain hidden sugar and salt.

[19] www.joslin.org, Joslin Diabetes Center. "Joslin Diabetes Center | Fitting Alcohol into Your Diabetic Meal Plan." *Fitting Alcohol into Your Diabetic Meal Plan | Joslin Diabetes Center,*
www.joslin.org/info/Fitting_Alcohol_Into_Your_Meal_Plan.html.
[20] "Reading Food Labels When You Have Diabetes." *WebMD,* WebMD, www.webmd.com/diabetes/how-read-food-labels#1.

Use this table to decipher part of the labels:

Label Claim	Definition (Standard Serving Size)
Fat-free or sugar-free	Less than 0.5 gram (g) of fat or sugar
Low fat	3 g of fat or less
Reduced fat or reduced sugar	At least 25% less fat or sugar than the regular product
Cholesterol free	Less than 2 milligrams (mg) cholesterol and 2g or less of saturated fat
Reduced cholesterol	At least 25% less cholesterol and 2 g or less of saturated fat
Calorie-free	Less than 5 calories
Low calorie	40 calories or less
Light	1/3 fewer calories or 50% less fat

Fact #6 – Benefits of Physical Activity

Physical exercise is one of the best ways to remain healthy by maintaining an adequate muscle mass, body weight, blood sugar range, and blood pressure; all of which are vital for maintaining sugar balance. Physical activity also improves blood circulation, the quality of your sleep, boosts your energy, elevates your mood, and promotes wellbeing.

Diabetics have a reduced muscle mass and are prone to imbalance. Your physical regimen should be customized to include walks, swimming, and weight training. Walks can be done just about anywhere. Start slowly 10 min at first if you have not exercised in a while working your way to at least 30 minutes daily, or a minimum of 150 minutes per week.[21] Add to your walk gentle stretching, basic yoga postures, swimming, and little weight training. The guiding principle here is to listen to your own body and increase the length and intensity of your physical activities, as you become accustomed to your exercise routine.

If you are at home convalescing after a hospital stay, it is best to start with light activities such as leg lifting, arm raising, and other range of motion exercises. You can also exercise while walking in place or around your house while doing light household chores. Consult with your doctor(s) and your support team to see which physical activities to incorporate into your daily routine. Similarly, if you are not convalescing, consult your doctor(s), your support team, and holistic practitioner to revise your care plan to include walks, swimming, and weight training in the privacy of your own home or at the gym.

---

[21] Colberg, Sheri R., et al. "Physical Activity/Exercise and Diabetes: A Position Statement of the American Diabetes Association." *Diabetes Care*, American Diabetes Association, 1 Nov. 2016, www.care.diabetesjournals.org/content/39/11/2065.

Apart from physical activities, breathing mindfully and getting enough sunlight can do wonders for your physical, mental, and emotional wellbeing. Deep breathing throughout the day at least 15-20 minutes of sunshine in the early morning and late afternoon are excellent for the mood, stress management, and absorption of natural Vitamin D, the sunshine vitamin. Some forms of meditation with the practice of pranayama, yoga breathing techniques, are also beneficial for inner peace, stress management, and building a stable emotional environment.

Be patient with yourself. It may take a while before the benefits of daily physical activity are visible and results are experienced. Change requires willpower and determination. Any additional therapeutic techniques such as hydrotherapy, massages, reflexology, aromatherapy, acupressure, and even relaxing with hobbies such as music, painting, or volunteering can support you in your achieving your goals and promote wellbeing.

Fact #7 – Managing Stress

Stress is a common factor leading to disease. Stress managed well has a positive effect on the body. However, unmanaged stress over a long time has a detrimental effect on your overall health. Stress overload can lead to developing many health conditions, including diabetes, due to the release of stress hormones like cortisol that raises blood sugar levels and promotes insulin resistance.

Stress is best managed with the support of friends and family members, your doctors and other health professionals, with physical and social activities, having a sense of purpose, taking care of yourself physically and emotionally, practicing introspection for self-awareness and helping others. The first step in managing stress is to identify what stress is, its effects on the body, what to do about it, and how to manage it.

"Stress is a physical and mental reaction to perceived danger. Conditions that are seen uncontrollable or require emotional and behavioral change tend to be perceived as a threat," according to Dr. Joseph Napora. Ph.D., LCSW-C.[22]

Stress can be harmful in many ways. It affects memory, triggers anxiety, negative emotions, poor eating habits, and often impairs the decision-making process and cognitive skills to name a few. Prolonged exposure to stress compromises the body's hormonal, immune, renal, digestive and reproductive systems, and may result in depression.

---

[22] "Managing Stress and Diabetes." *American Diabetes Association*, www.diabetes.org/living-with-diabetes/parents-and-kids/everyday-life/managing-stress-and-diabetes.html.

Stress affects each person differently. Common signs and symptoms associated with stress are sleeping too much or too little, eating too much or too little, weight loss or gain, muscle loss, increased heart rate and loss of self-esteem, which can lead to depression.

Creative hobbies such as reading, writing, positive thinking, meditation, visualization, and therapy for emotional and physical distress are all effective ways to manage stress. Being mindful that these activities have the power to heal you of stress and empower you to live a normal healthy life.

Stress management decreases insulin sensitivity, lower insulin requirements, and keeps blood glucose stable. Reading and writing are therapeutic activities and can redirect the mind to be more productive and promote healing.

Positive thinking and the practice of introspection through meditation have been known to lower stress as well as blood pressure. Both help to maintain hormonal and emotional balance. Being able to sit in silence and let go of daily stressors promote the release of feel-good hormones that lower blood glucose levels. In turn, the body can heal.

Adopting a mindful attitude towards life by paying attention to your thoughts, feelings, and actions is a great approach to overcome lifestyle choices that no longer serve you while adopting habits that promote a healthier you.

Taking the time to sit in silence to discover yourself and reflect on who you are can lead to self-awareness, which helps you to relax and conquer harmful stressors and fears. Self-discovery will also empower you to take charge as you progress in your journey and find answers as to why you do what you do and what is causing you to act or feel a certain way.

Unresolved angst and fears may cause depression, physical and mental fatigue. If you have diabetes, you are at greater risk of suffering from depression as you may not only feel isolated and overwhelmed by your condition but may also suffer from hormonal imbalance. The reverse is also true. Patients who suffer from depression have an increased risk of developing Type 2 diabetes. Stress management is of paramount importance. Both conditions can be tackled at the same time.

Common means of relieving symptoms of depression include social and physical activity, participating in hobbies, sports, games, yoga and music therapy, reflexology, acupuncture, healthy eating habits, and weight to name a few. The same activities are also beneficial for managing your condition. The two conditions are intertwined.

The term *diapression* = *diabetes* + *depression* has been coined by Dr. Paul Ciechanowski to describe specific characteristics observed in people suffering from both diabetes and depression where the symptoms of diabetes are aggravated by depression. Depression is apparent in poor self-care behavior and results in the inadequate management of the condition.[23]

---

[23] Ciechanowski, Paul. "Diapression: An Integrated Model for Understanding the Experience of Individuals with Co-Occurring Diabetes and Depression." *Clinical Diabetes*, American Diabetes Association, 1 Apr. 2011, clinical.diabetesjournals.org/content/29/2/43.

Fact #8 – Managing Cholesterol

According to Mayo Clinic, lifestyle changes are essential to improving your lipid values, also known as cholesterol levels, which include HDL, LDL, and triglycerides. In particular, efforts should be made to keep your LDL below 100mg/dL as lowering your LDL will reduce the probability of heart disease.

Keeping your numbers within range will most likely require some lifestyle changes such as losing excess weight, eating healthier foods, and increasing your physical activity. You should also discuss the consumption of alcohol with your endocrinologist and your support system. If you smoke, it is recommended that you quit. The latter cannot be stressed enough.

Smoking is especially detrimental to your health. It aggravates your condition and associated complications by damaging the walls of your blood vessels, making them more prone to fatty deposits accumulation. It may also impact your HDL, or "good cholesterol" by lowering it. All of this should be kept in mind when tracking your cholesterol LDL and HDL levels, and your very-low-density lipoprotein (VLDL) levels. [24]

The Mayo Clinic has published the below guidelines to interpret lipid values. You can use those to better understand your numbers and to have targeted conversations with your doctors, dietician or nutritionist, holistic practitioner, and other health professionals.

---

[24] "High Cholesterol." *Mayo Clinic*, Mayo Foundation for Medical Education and Research, 23 Feb. 2019, www.mayoclinic.org/diseases-conditions/high-blood-cholesterol/symptoms-causes/syc-20350800.

In addition to factors such as eating habits and smoking, which can lower your HDL and contribute to having high cholesterol, your genetic makeup and age play a role as well.

Total cholesterol (U.S. & some other countries)	Total cholesterol (Canada & most of Europe)*	
Below 200 mg/dL	Below 5.2 mmol/L	Desirable
200-239 mg/dL	5.2-6.2 mmol/L	Borderline high
240 mg/dL & above	Above 6.2 mmol/L	High

Triglycerides (U.S. & some other countries)	Triglycerides (Canada & most of Europe)*	
Below 150 mg/dL	Below 1.7 mmol/L	Desirable
150-199 mg/dL	1.7-2.2 mmol/L	Borderline high
200-499 mg/dL	2.3-5.6 mmol/L	High
500 mg/dL and above	Above 5.6 mmol/L	Very high

LDL cholesterol (U.S. and some other countries)	LDL cholesterol (Canada and most of Europe)*	
Below 70 mg/dL	Below 1.8 mmol/L	Best for people who have heart disease or diabetes.
Below 100 mg/dL	Below 2.6 mmol/L	Optimal for people at risk of heart disease.
100-129 mg/dL	2.6-3.3 mmol/L	Near-optimal if there is no heart disease. High if there is heart disease.
130-159 mg/dL	3.4-4.1 mmol/L	Borderline high if there is no heart disease. High if there is heart disease.
160-189 mg/dL	4.1-4.9 mmol/L	High if there is no heart disease. Very high if there is heart disease.

HDL cholesterol (U.S and some other countries)	HDL cholesterol (Canada and most of Europe)*	
Below 40 mg/dL, men Below 50 mg/dL, women	Below 1 mmol/L Below 1.3 mmol/L	Poor
40-59 mg/dL, men 50-59 mg/dL, women	1-1.5 mmol/L 1.3-1.5 mmol/L	Better
60 mg/dL and above	Above 1.5 mmol/L	Best

Note: Canadian and European cholesterol and triglycerides guidelines differ slightly from U.S. guidelines. These conversions are based on U.S. guidelines. [25]

[25] "High Cholesterol." *Mayo Clinic*, Mayo Foundation for Medical Education and Research, 15 Aug. 2017, www.mayoclinic.org/diseases-conditions/high-blood-cholesterol/diagnosis-treatment/drc-20350806.

Fact #9 – Aging and Type 2 Diabetes

As we age, the chances of acquiring Type 2 diabetes, or adult-onset diabetes, increases. The body becomes more resistant to insulin or the pancreas may stop producing enough insulin. Therefore, as we advance in years, you must adopt a healthy lifestyle, work on our emotional triggers, and follow a disciplined approach.

There is no point in having insulin, then yield to the constant temptations of consuming unhealthy food and sugary drinks that make your blood sugar spike. Besides, excess weight or obesity, inactivity or sedentary life, and poor lifestyle choices have all contributed to the onset of your condition and are particularly detrimental now as shown in this book.

While other factors may lead to the onset of diabetes such as a gene mutation (or MODY) as we get older, you can still avoid complications by following your endocrinologist's plan of care, using a diary to record your food and medication intake, and partaking in physical activities. The diary is especially important, as it will help you and your support team to identify your progress, the behaviors and triggers you may want to work on and the goals you want to achieve.

It is also true that we cannot stop the aging clock. Yet remaining active and immediately reporting any concerns to your doctors can prevent any exacerbations; avoid E.R. and hospital visits, which are all essential to living a healthy life.

Aging and diabetes can affect your body in many ways:

Eye problems — cataracts, glaucoma, and retinopathy can be exacerbated with uncontrolled diabetes. See your eye doctor yearly.

Gum diseases — you can be more prone to infections. Be diligent with your oral care, brushing and flossing daily. Schedule regular six months cleaning with your dentist.

Falls — neuropathy is nerve damage caused by hyperglycemia and uncontrolled diabetes. This condition causes pain, numbness in the feet and hands and tingling sensation. If you experience less sensation in your feet, you may be more prone to frequent falls. Also, examine your feet daily for any wounds.

Flu and pneumonia — if you are over 65, it is very important to have your regular vaccines to prevent risks of serious complications from decreased immunity. Pneumonia, bronchitis, sinus infections, and ear infections are common and often treated successfully. They can, however, be deadly to persons with a compromised immune system with diabetes.

Fact #10 – Finding Out More …

Learning does not stop with this book. It is a continuous process. There is a lot of information published on the internet, magazines, and medical journals about your condition.

You can consult these sources to educate yourself further, to better understand your condition and any other health setbacks that you may be experiencing. You can also read about new habits that you can incorporate in your daily routine or simply find delicious meal plans online specifically designed for your condition, and much more. You may join a support group to share your thoughts and for emotional support.

Listed below are a few agencies and medical schools that publish articles on Type 2 diabetes, stress management, healthy diet, physical exercises, quitting smoking, and other health topics.

While this is not a comprehensive list by any means, it is an excellent start. You can either go directly to the website to research various topics or call to request more information:

American Diabetes Association
1-800-342-2383 (toll-free)
Email: askada@diabetes.org
Website: www.diabetes.org

American Heart Association
1-800-AHA-USA-1 or 1-800-242-8721
Outside of the US: +1-214-570-5978
Website: www.heart.org

American Stroke Association
1-800-AHA-USA-1 or 1-800-242-8721
Outside of the US: +1-214-570-5978
Website: www.strokeassociation.org

Centers for Disease Control and Prevention (CDC)
1-800-232-4636 (toll-free)
1-888-232-6348 (TTY/toll-free)
Email: cdcinfo@cdc.gov
Website: www.cdc.gov

Cleveland Clinic
Website: www.health.clevelandclinic.org

Diabetes Education Online
1-415-353-2266
Website: www.dtc.ucsf.edu

Diabetes Care Program | Stanford Health Care
1-650-498-900
Website: www.stanfordhealthcare.org

Harvard Health Publishing
Harvard Medical School
Website: www.health.harvard.edu

Joslin Diabetes Center
1-617-309-2400
Website: www.joslin.org

The National Cancer Institute's Smoking Quitline
1-877-448-7848
1-877-44U-QUIT/toll-free
Email: cancergovstaff@mail.nih.gov

The National Institute of Diabetes, Digestive, and Kidney Diseases (NIDDK)
1-800-874-8747 (toll-free)
1-866-569-1162 (TTY/toll-free)
Email: healthinfo@niddk.nih.gov
Website: www.niddk.nih.gov

Mayo Clinic
By state: www.mayoclinic.org/about-mayo-clinic/contact/
By condition: www.mayoclinic.org/diseases-conditions/diabetes/

Smokefree 60+
Website: www.60plus.smokefree.gov

Fact # 11 – Meaningful Dialogues with Doctors

Reflecting on the content of this book, what meaningful conversations can you have with your doctor(s), endocrinologist, and other members of your support team that would be the most beneficial to you?

Earlier on in this book, you learned that it is medically proven that nutrition, diet, physical exercise, stress management, and emotional stability apart from medications can affect your condition positively or adversely. As such, all those must be evaluated thoroughly to be either modified, left as is, or incorporated as part of your daily life if you are to keep your diabetes and other chronic conditions under control. Like many chronic conditions, Type 2 diabetes requires lifestyle changes that are primarily achievable by monitoring your vital signs and keeping track of everything you eat, your medication intake and physical activity as a part of your daily life.

Self-discipline, perseverance, and determination to work towards achieving these/your goals are necessary to delay, mitigate, and/or prevent complications from your condition. While it can be hard to remain motivated, do not give up! You are not alone.

It is important to watch your mood and to share your feelings with your support system, especially if feeling overwhelmed, anxious about your condition or if you experience any form of distress such as lack of sleep, irritability, mood swings to name a few. Many diabetics suffer from *diapression*.

Throughout the book, we have continuously stressed the importance of record-keeping as illustrated in the sample log at the end of the book, or a companion diary, and how keeping a record of those results will help you have meaningful dialogues with your endocrinologist and your support team, which is an integral part of your care.

A companion diary will not only help you achieve your goals, potentially avoiding complications, but can also make it easier for you to live a healthier, joyful life while keeping your condition under control. Remember the companion diary, while helpful to you, is to be essentially used by your doctor(s) and endocrinologist to carry out a systematic review of your condition as part of a holistic individualized patient care framework, so do not forget to take it with you to your appointments. Having the daily logs handy ensure that the information being discussed is complete and accurate.

This approach will make it easier for you to notice any behavioral changes, blood sugar level changes, and other changes that should be reviewed with doctors and vice versa. Prevention and preventive measures are to be emphasized here. The approach is instrumental in prioritizing the topics to be discussed with your doctor(s). As a tool, a companion diary contains the baseline information needed to better understand your condition. Therefore, it is best used to facilitate conversations with your support team, especially when meeting with your doctor(s).

At this point, if you compare your understanding of your condition now as opposed to before reading this book, which changes can you make to improve the quality of your life?

Would these changes include both keeping a daily log and working diligently and patiently towards achieving the goals you set for yourself, which are of utmost importance for your continuous progress towards managing your condition and keeping your diabetes under control?

Are you willing to have candid discussions with your support team and endocrinologist about your progress and any concerns you may have? Are you able to see yourself making those changes? Do you need help from your doctors to implement any or all changes? Can your current support team help? Or, do you need to enlist others?

If so, take action now! Set up an appointment with your endocrinologist to discuss your condition and your goals. Also, be sure to schedule the required medical tests and exams for this year.

Fact #12 – Scheduling Medical Examination & Diagnostics

Several diagnostics and physical examinations are needed to monitor and manage your condition in addition to a complete blood count (CBC) and urine test that your primary care physician may order as part of your annual physical exam.

The following guidelines may be used by you for your investigations and in consultation with your doctor:

Tests or Exams	Date	Next
HbA1c or Hemoglobin A1c – a quarterly test to evaluate the average amount of glucose in your bloodstream over the last 2 to 3 months (see HbA1c chart).		
Lipid Profile or Lipid Panel – an annual or as needed panel of blood tests that serves as an initial screening tool for abnormalities in lipids, such as cholesterol and triglycerides.		
Blood Pressure Tests – an annual or as needed. This may include several tests to help your doctor(s) choose the right lifestyle changes and medicines for you to lower your blood pressure. Your doctor may want to see if your blood pressure has affected your body and its organs.		

Blood Urea Nitrogen (BUN), Urine Albumin (aka. microalbumin) and Creatinine – an annual test or as needed to check for kidney disease…		
Kidney Function Test (KFT) – an annual test or as needed to determine how well the kidneys are functioning.		
Dental exam – regular semi-annual visits are important to check the overall health of your gums and teeth, which can improve blood sugar control.		
Retinal Exam – an annual exam is important. Diabetes can lead to vision loss (blindness) if not kept under control. Diabetic retinopathy is caused by damage to the blood vessels in the tissue at the back of the eye (retina). A diabetic retinopathy exam can help preserve your eyesight.		
Foot Exam- an annual exam is important. Diabetic neuropathy causes nerve damages and reduces sensation. Injuries or infected wounds can lead to amputation.		
Notes		

Fact #13 – Lessons to Be Learned with a 12-Week Program

While most diabetics are aware of the importance of keeping track of their numbers, what we hear most often is that "keeping a record is hard and knowing what to keep track of is even harder."

That is no longer a challenge, as we have done the work for you by providing the necessary education, raising awareness of potential complications, and designing a companion diary to this book that is easy to use and allows for daily recording of the essentials.

So, why 12-week? Which lessons can you expect to learn?

Letting go of old habits and forming new habits take a while. Keeping a 12-week daily log helps you to track and monitor progress to manage your condition systematically over a specific period. Patterns and progress become easier to detect, more visible. Summarizing those at the end of each week is also useful. The extra step forces you to make a conscious effort to review your past entries, reflect on your accomplishments, and choose your goal(s) for the following week. This step is the equivalent of *Reflection Page* in the companion diary.

While you continuously monitor your progress and review your goals, your awareness of your condition and overall health will increase. Some patterns will become clearer. You will develop a better understanding of your daily habits, emotional triggers, and stressors. You will also know whether you are on track or need to make further lifestyle changes and/or medication adjustments. You will begin to see what works and does not work for you, making it easier for you to form healthier habits and forgo others.

In setting your weekly or monthly goals, be sure to employ a S.M.A.R.T (specific, measurable, actionable, realistic, and timely) approach. Discuss your goals with your doctors and support team as often as you can. Your holistic practitioner, if you have enlisted one, can also help you identify and refine your goals further as part of your individualized care plan.

This 12-week daily framework is of paramount importance. It allows you and your support team to track and make the necessary changes and tweaks gradually throughout your journey, often increasing your chances of keeping your diabetes under control while delaying, mitigating, and/or preventing complications from your condition.

Diligently recording all daily activities for 12-week is the foundation for a healthier you. At the end of the process, you can judge for yourself, which lifestyle changes work best for you and what other goals you may want to set for yourself. The companion diary to this book is also conveniently designed to track your progress quarterly, which is the same timeframe used for HbA1c monitoring.

As previously mentioned, HbA1c is a quarterly test that evaluates the average amount of glucose in your bloodstream over the last 2 to 3 months. Therefore, you can continue to use copies of the companion diary for as long as it is needed to achieve the best possible results while following the guidelines outlined in this book.

If you are already keeping a diary of your design, consider looking at the entries for this week and noting what stands out:

_____
_____
_____
_____
_____
_____
_____

Use this opportunity to go over the habits you want to keep as well and document why:

_____
_____
_____
_____

Similarly, document the habits and behaviors you want to work on. What are those? Why do you want to change them? Do you need help? Can you ask your support team for guidance?

_____
_____
_____
_____
_____
_____
_____

Do not forget to highlight all the progress you have made to date:

_____
_____
_____
_____

In addition, which achievements are you the proudest of?

_____
_____
_____
_____

Additional comments:

_____
_____

Fact #14 – Main Guidelines for a Diabetic Patient

In this endeavor, the most important person is you. The main guidelines for a diabetic patient are:

- ☐ Educate yourself about your condition
- ☐ Work out a support system
- ☐ Revisit your support system as needed
- ☐ Opt for a holistic approach
- ☐ Use a diary or daily log to record:
  - Vital signs (blood sugar levels and blood pressure)
  - Wounds if any
  - Food & medication intake
  - Physical activities
- ☐ Use the same diary to:
  - Reflect on your mood, i.e. mental and emotional health
  - Forgo behaviors that do not promote a healthier you and adopt new ones
  - Review progress before, during, and after medical appointments
- ☐ Do not run out of supplies:
  - Test three times daily if you are on insulin
  - Daily, and as needed, if you are on an oral anti-diabetic medication
- ☐ Make healthy dietary choices
- ☐ Avoid consumption of tobacco and sugar-based beverages
- ☐ Maintain a balanced body weight
- ☐ Perform some physical activity regularly
- ☐ Manage stress, especially emotional stress
- ☐ Have regular screening and diagnosis
- ☐ Aim to keep your diabetes under control to delay, mitigate, and/or prevent complications!

Conclusion

If you have come thus far, congratulations! You are now aware of the most important and latest facts related to your condition, Type 2 diabetes. You also know how to actively keep track of your condition by following the guidelines included in this book. You can utilize its resources to significantly improve the quality of your life, and your chances of managing adequately your condition to bring your diabetes under control, keep the same condition under control and delay, mitigate, and/or prevent complications.

This book includes the latest research currently available to us to ensure that you have full awareness of your condition. We also sought input from Dr. Narottam Bharadwaj, a world-renowned diabetes specialist who has dedicated the past forty years to the study of this condition and author of the foreword.

Going back to pre-diabetes, a potentially reversible and preventable condition, we have shown that this condition is the initial manifestation of the onset of the disease. Also, the same preventable pre-diabetic condition will most likely lead to diabetes if left unchecked. The main culprit for pre-diabetes is obesity; a risk factor, which continues to be prevalent amongst those suffering this condition, Type 2 diabetes.

From there, we have established that once the condition manifests itself, keeping a daily log of all activities and periodically reviewing your records with your support team, especially your endocrinologist, is an essential part of your care to manage your condition. Similarly, a strong support system that enlists the help of the trusted friend(s), family member(s), doctors and other professionals will ensure the best results. A holistic approach is, therefore, best suited to address your needs and your condition.

At the same time, you need to have the will power and desire to gradually improve your condition, namely your sugar levels, cholesterol, and blood pressure, through lifestyle changes apart from taking medications. A holistic practitioner can help you put together such an individualized care plan while coordinating with your healthcare team.

Keeping a diary or daily log that contains a record of all your activities, including all you eat daily over a given period, such as 12 weeks or 90 days, is not only a powerful tool but is also a practical, sensible tool. In addition, this diary should include the medications and time when they were administered and any form of physical activity you performed. Those have been detailed in the companion diary that you can purchase for yourself.

Being aware of all your daily activities is of vital importance. It will help you make significant and long-lasting lifestyle changes so that you can live life to its fullest and "age gracefully." Stress management is quintessential to maintain hormonal balance and avoid further complications from your condition and a myriad of other diseases, including depression, high blood pressure, and coronary artery disease as has been covered adequately in this book.

With the help of your support team, any lifestyle changes you make will be instrumental in managing your condition and in delaying, mitigating, or preventing potential health complications related to Type 2 diabetes. These lifestyle changes will assist you in living a healthier life with your condition.

You can use this book to educate yourself and the companion diary to maintain records essential to manage and review your condition with your doctors and support team. You can also review your daily records to …:

- Reflect on what matters the most to you to live a happier healthier life
- Set goals for yourself and review them with your support team
- Identify triggers that lead to a spike in blood sugar levels, cholesterol, and blood pressure

Your support system can help you achieve your goals and live a healthier life. Remember to do your part to achieve your goals. You are not alone. 422 million people have one form of diabetes. Make a choice today to be a fighter to improve the quality of your life.

If you purchase the companion diary to this book, you can begin right away. The diary will allow you to record daily activities pertinent to your condition and to keep track of your progress for 12 weeks or 90 days for a systematic review by your endocrinologist and other doctors from time-to-time. You will also be able to reflect on your goals and share your progress and concerns with your entire support team.

The diary includes a short introduction, a page to transcribe the names of your support team, record upcoming appointments, daily logs, and reflection pages. Why not take advantage now?

This is the link to purchase, or go to Amazon:

The Companion Diary to *Three Steps: Track, Manage Type 2 Diabetes & Prevent Complications!*

In addition to the above, as previously noted, a holistic practitioner can help you put together an individualized plan to manage your condition and organize aspects of your care requiring primarily your attention such as close monitoring of daily activities, stress management, nutrition, and physical activities.

At the same time, the holistic practitioner can coordinate with your doctors and support team to deliver the best results. Do not wait any longer, see the sample log!

Sample Log

WEEK 1 – Tuesday: 1/1/2019			☺ What is your mood today?

<table>
<tr><td colspan="3" align="center">Vital Signs</td><td align="center">Food Log</td></tr>
<tr><td>Blood Sugar</td><td>Time</td><td>Level</td><td></td></tr>
<tr><td>Fasting (a.m.)</td><td>10 a.m.</td><td>98</td><td>Meals Taken | Time</td></tr>
<tr><td>Random</td><td>5p.m.</td><td>100</td><td>Breakfast   8 a.m.</td></tr>
<tr><td>Blood pressure</td><td></td><td></td><td>1 egg, 1 whole-wheat toast, 1 cup of fruits,</td></tr>
<tr><td>Morning (a.m.)</td><td>10 a.m.</td><td>120/80</td><td>almond milk, and hot tea.</td></tr>
<tr><td>Random</td><td>5 p.m.</td><td>135/90</td><td>Blood sugar 1 or 2 hours after (optional) 150</td></tr>
<tr><td>Wounds</td><td colspan="2">Check your feet!</td><td></td></tr>
<tr><td colspan="3">Describe your wounds here:

No wounds
Skin intact
No blisters
No callus (to be shaved off)
Or, small wound under toes</td><td>Snack   10 a.m.
1 cup of fruits

Lunch   12 a.m. or p.m.
½ cup of soup, 1/2 avocado, 1 green salad with
nuts and chicken, 1 whole-wheat toast.
Blood sugar 1 or 2 hours after (optional) 130</td></tr>
<tr><td colspan="3" align="center">Medication Log & Blood Sugar before meals,
including Insulin</td><td>Snack   3 p.m.
1 unsweetened yogurt, blueberries</td></tr>
<tr><td colspan="3">Morning (Time/Dosage)   Blood Sugar 98
500 mg of metformin
Insulin per sliding scale</td><td>Dinner   9 p.m.
1 piece of salmon, 1 sweet potatoes, Brussels
sprouts
Blood sugar 1 or 2 hours after (optional) 145</td></tr>
<tr><td colspan="3">Lunch (Time/Dosage)   Blood Sugar 98
500 mg of metformin</td><td>Snack   ———
p.m.
1 piece of fresh string cheese</td></tr>
<tr><td colspan="3">Dinner (Time/Dosage)   Blood Sugar 110
500 mg of metformin</td><td align="center">Activity Log</td></tr>
<tr><td colspan="3"></td><td>Describe your activities here:
X 10 min ___ min   Water intake
___ miles or ___ steps ___ Oz or 8 Glasses</td></tr>
<tr><td colspan="4">Notes: I am feeling generalized pain on and off</td></tr>
</table>

HbA1c or Hemoglobin A1c Test

Commonly used to diagnose Type 1 and Type 2 diabetes, the HbA1c test measures the average blood sugar (glucose) level over 2-3 months. The same test is used to monitor how well you are managing your diabetes.

This test is not a substitute for self-monitoring. Daily self-monitoring allows you to see how your daily activities affect your blood sugar. You can then opt to make healthier choices. Keep in mind that a normal A1c level for someone, who does not have diabetes, is below 5.7 percent. A range from 5.7 and 6.4 percent indicates pre-diabetes (i.e. impaired fasting glucose) with a high risk of developing diabetes later on.

An A1c level of 6.5 percent or higher on two separate tests shows that you are diabetics. Above 8 percent, your diabetes is not properly managed. You are at a higher risk of developing complications. Your doctor(s) and support team can work with you to keep your diabetes under control.

The recommended target is an A1c level of 7 percent or less for diabetics. This percentage can be lower or higher for some individuals according to the Mayo Clinic. If your A1c level is above the recommended target, your doctor(s) may revise your diabetes treatment plan to better manage your condition and prevent complications.

The Mayo clinic also points out that A1c results may not be accurate for those who have a hemoglobin variant. Your doctor(s) can further advise..[26]

---

[26] "A1C Test." *Mayo Clinic*, Mayo Foundation for Medical Education and Research, 18 Dec. 2018, www.mayoclinic.org/tests-procedures/a1c-test/about/pac-20384643.

The tables below show how to interpret your A1c levels:

A1c level	Estimated average blood sugar level	Meaning
5.7 percent	**117mg/dL (6.5 mmol/L)**	**Below 5.7%, no diabetes**
6 percent	126 mg/dL (7 mmol/L)	Between 5.7 and 6.4 indicates pre-diabetes
6.4 percent	137 mg/dl (7.6 mmol/L)	
6.5 percent	**140 mg/dl (7.7 mmol/L)**	**6.5% or higher on two separate tests indicates diabetes**
7 percent	154 mg/dL (8.6 mmol/L)	7% or less is the recommended A1c target for most diabetics

A1c level	Estimated average blood sugar level	Meaning
8 percent	**183 mg/dL (10.2 mmol/L)**	**8% or higher, your diabetes is not managed properly.**
9 percent	212 mg/dL (11.8 mmol/L)	
10 percent	240 mg/dL (13.4 mmol/L)	
11 percent	269 mg/dL (14.9 mmol/L)	
12 percent	298 mg/dL (16.5 mmol/L)	
13 percent	326 mg/dL (18 mmol/L)	
14 percent	355 mg/dL (19.7 mmol/L)	

About the Authors

Drawing from traditional holistic practices (complementary medicine) and the latest medical research (modern medicine), Samya and Sandra have co-authored this book to help those suffering from Type 2 diabetes learn important facts about their condition and how daily monitoring can improve your chances of keeping your condition under control and living a healthy and blissful life. If you work diligently with the help of your endocrinologist and support team, you can delay, mitigate, and/or prevent complications related to your condition.

Samya is a holistic practitioner and private care manager in California, where she lives with her husband. She is also a certified yoga master, meditation teacher, and author of books and presentations on topics that complement allopathic treatments to help improve the quality of life of those receiving care. She is a frequent guest speaker at the Zuckerberg San Francisco General Hospital Wellness Center for the C.A.R.E (Cancer Awareness, Resources, and Education) program. Samya holds an M.A. and other health-related certifications.

Sandra is a registered home health director of patient care services and practices as a registered nurse in California, where she lives with her husband and children. She owned and managed Five Stars Alternative Care Nursing homes in the Midwest for a decade. Sandra is an avid meditation practitioner belonging to Self-Realization Fellowship.